"A great book on how men, how all of us, can connect through vulnerability and grow together."

Russell Brand

"A beautifully brave book by a very modern-day human. In Man Down, *Charlie Hoare stands naked in front of the macho all-boy's club of life and opens his heart. With solid advice and simple tips, Charlie invites culturally handcuffed men all over the world to own their emotions and talk about how they feel.*"

Ed Stafford

"A wise, compassionate, clear and ultimately helpful guide to the struggles many men face, gently offering constructive ways to be kinder to ourselves, to reach out for help, to heal our wounds and to live the best life we can."

Dr Tim Lomas, Senior Lecturer in Positive Psychology, University of East London

MAN DOWN

An Hachette UK Company
www.hachette.co.uk

Vie Books, an imprint of Summersdale Publishers Ltd
Part of Octopus Publishing Group Limited
Carmelite House
50 Victoria Embankment
LONDON
EC4Y 0DZ
UK

www.summersdale.com

Printed and bound in the Czech Republic

ISBN: 978-1-78783-250-3

Substantial discounts on bulk quantities of Summersdale books are available to corporations, professional associations and other organizations. For details contact general enquiries: telephone: +44 (0) 1243 771107 or email: enquiries@summersdale.com.

Disclaimer
The information given in this book should not be treated as a substitute for qualified medical advice. Neither the author nor the publisher can be held responsible for any loss or claim arising out of the use, or misuse, of the suggestions made or the failure to take medical advice.

MAN DOWN

A Guide for Men on Mental Health

CHARLIE HOARE

For Pip

CONTENTS

INTRODUCTION

Like many other men, on the surface it looks like I have life pretty sorted. At the age of 36 I've got a wonderful partner, a baby on the way, a house, a supportive family and friends. I've lived and worked abroad for five years, completed a dream trip of cycling 10,000 miles from Malaysia to London, co-founded a business and been back to university to study for a master's degree in positive psychology.

But underneath this "successful" exterior I'm a man with deep insecurities and anxieties that prevent me from sleeping more than five hours per night, connecting with others and generally enjoying life. You might question why someone with these sorts of issues is qualified to advise; but having experienced mental health disorders, had professional help and tried a lot of alternative coping strategies, I have learned lessons, some of which may be of use to you.

The biggest learning through my mental health journey has been the importance of opening up. It's so easy to say and so hard to do, but talking to your friends, family or colleagues is the best step you can take to improving how you feel. In recent years, I have opened up about my mental health challenges and shared vulnerabilities from my past, such as how I had a tough time at school, being bullied both physically and emotionally. I worried that people would reject me, but in fact I have found the complete opposite, with others empathizing and sharing their own life challenges.

So much has been done to reduce the stigma around mental health and we are slowly redefining what it means to be a man, but there is still a long way to go. According to the World Health Organization (WHO), at the time of writing the global suicide rate is a staggering one person every 40 seconds, and twice as many suicides are male, perhaps principally because men are less likely to ask for help. So why not try having some deeper conversations with your friends? Show some vulnerability about how you're feeling and see how they respond. This book is written to enable you to do exactly that – by helping you to understand what mental health really is, and showing you that it's totally normal to discuss how you're feeling.

Courage starts with showing up and letting ourselves be seen.

BRENÉ BROWN

CHAPTER 1

MAN UP — WHAT'S THE PROBLEM?

So why are some men so bad at connecting with their emotions and opening up about their mental health? We learn (potentially harmful) habits and beliefs through our cultures and societies about how we should behave. We look to male role models, perhaps men close to us, or men in the media, and follow their example. It's time to challenge some of those behaviours and beliefs for the sake of the mental health of men everywhere.

TRADITIONAL MASCULINITY IN A MODERN WORLD

My perception of the traditional narrative around masculinity is that boys have to be tough, taking life's adversities on the chin, not showing weakness. This conventional view that masculinity is about strength, courage and independence perhaps worked in the distant past, when we had to be the protectors and hunters for our species, but in the modern world these traits are purely admirable, not essential, particularly when you are doing yourself harm to maintain them.

In reality, it wasn't beneficial for me to be what I thought was courageous in the face of bullying, trying to avoid showing weakness by not admitting it to anyone. In fact, trying to live up to these perceived masculine ideals only prolonged and worsened my situation, as no one knew I needed help. Being vulnerable is being human, and having the courage to admit weakness is a sign of strength in your character.

THE PRIVILEGE OF A LIFETIME IS TO BECOME WHO YOU TRULY ARE.

CARL JUNG

"DON'T EXPRESS YOURSELF"

As men, at least in Western societies, we're often described as not being in touch with our feelings like women are. Because of the way we are generally socialized with masculine stereotyping from a young age, our ability to deal with emotions has been consistently undermined. There's actually a term for this in psychology – normative male alexithymia – which defines a situation where the way that men are brought up to behave in society conflicts with the emotions that they feel and express.

This totally fits with my own experience, having grown up believing that men don't have feelings like women do. But this is absolute nonsense; men, women and, in fact, humans with any gender identity feel emotions equally; the problem is that men are encouraged not to show them. I think some of us suppress our feelings so much that we don't even realize that we're doing it. I've spent most of my life repressing my emotions so that I can present what I think is the "correct" or "socially acceptable" version of myself to the world – regardless of how I've felt. Perhaps you can identify with this?

"TAKE IT LIKE A MAN"

Every guy can relate to being told to "be a man about it" or "take it like a man". Being tough and getting on with life can be a useful strategy sometimes, but sometimes it can be damaging. It's so important to be open about what you're going through. Not opening up about being bullied and repressing all the negative emotions that went along with that had long-term adverse consequences for my mental health. I have spent 20 years trying to undo and manage the resulting trauma.

Can you think of times where you've had to take an experience "like a man", despite knowing that it's damaging you? You might be holding on to that negative experience, but with time you can learn to release the unexpressed emotions and unburden yourself.

"This is one of the challenges of masculinity, as admitting to having a mental health problem is often wrongly viewed by men as admitting weakness."

SANE, mental health charity

"BOYS DON'T CRY"

As men we're generally not encouraged to be open with our thoughts and feelings. I remember frequently locking myself in the toilet at school and crying my eyes out – it was the only safe space I could find to get away, be vulnerable and feel better. Crying is a totally normal reaction to negative emotions and is a natural response by the body to improve your state of mind by activating the parasympathetic nervous system (aiding relaxation) and releasing oxytocin and endorphins (improving your mood). In fact, if you don't let yourself feel these negative emotions, then you will carry that negative energy instead of releasing it.

Have you ever noticed how you feel so much better after you have let yourself cry? I now want to cry more than I am able to! I'm learning how to get in touch with my emotions. So if you feel like crying, let it all out. Your body and mind will thank you for it.

Boys don't cry,
but men do.

MALORIE BLACKMAN

THE ALPHA MALE

Our society has traditionally celebrated the "alpha male" – the most successful and powerful male in a group who likes to be in charge of others. Men who are dominant and limit their emotional range primarily to expressions of anger have been the holders of power and wealth for centuries. Studies of social animals have shown that individuals exhibiting alpha traits gain preferential access to food and sex. Luckily, qualities that are less "alpha", such as empathy, are being celebrated in modern society, but the underlying natural bias toward alpha males remains. When extroverted, competitive, unemotional males are celebrated by our culture, it's difficult for men who don't fit that image to express themselves authentically.

Try not to become a man of success, but rather try to become a man of value.

ALBERT EINSTEIN

THE BETA MALE

Men who don't show the classic alpha male characteristics are often labelled as "beta males". This is a term which has historically been used to describe men who are largely submissive, passive or subservient, all traits with arguably negative connotations in mainstream culture. So it's no surprise that many of us, including myself, have tried to portray alpha traits despite feeling much more beta inside. It seems to me that more recent positive descriptions of the beta side of the male persona, such as being sensitive and emotionally intelligent, are helping to improve perceptions of men who don't exhibit the traditionally revered alpha tendencies.

HUMAN FIRST

Why is not expressing emotions often viewed to be "acting like a man"? Perhaps we need to move away entirely from old-fashioned notions of masculine and feminine. Humans experience a wide range of emotions so why do we feel the need to assign a gender stereotype to them?

THIS IS THE SCRIPT THAT WE'VE BEEN GIVEN: GIRLS ARE WEAK, AND BOYS ARE STRONG...

THIS IS TOXIC AND HAS TO END.

JUSTIN BALDONI

It can affect anyone

Just like nasty physical diseases like cancer, mental health conditions can strike anyone at any time. As with cancer, there are factors that can increase your risk of suffering from anxiety or depression such as bereavement, job loss or relationship breakdown. Ignoring the problem won't make it go away. True strength comes from acknowledging that you are struggling and making attempts to manage how you are feeling.

TURN YOUR WOUNDS INTO WISDOM.

OPRAH WINFREY

A TOTALLY NORMAL PROBLEM

At the time of writing, research estimates that one in six people in the past week experienced a common mental health problem. According to WHO, one in four people in the world will be affected by a mental health condition at some point in their lives and two in three people never seek help from a health professional.

Mental health is simply a part of life, just as physical health is. It's normal to have the flu or a rash or a hole in your tooth, just as it is normal to have ups and downs mentally. The key is to recognize and manage the symptoms of the flu to prevent it from turning into full-blown pneumonia. Ideally, we protect ourselves from becoming mentally ill in the first place but, as with our physical health, we know that this is not always possible, despite our best efforts.

GUILT OF FEELING LOW

Sometimes you have a clear reason to feel depressed or anxious – perhaps you've lost your job, broken up with your partner or someone close to you has passed away – but it's also totally acceptable to feel down when everything in your life is seemingly going well.

There may be genetic predispositions in your family, you may be suffering from hormonal imbalances, your diet might be affecting how you feel or it could be something else entirely. Sometimes you feel bad and don't know why. This is OK! As men, we often feel that we're meant to be the strong ones, so we can feel particularly guilty for feeling down when everything looks rosy on the outside. Accepting how you are feeling is the first step to managing your mental health.

Acceptance doesn't mean resignation; it means understanding that something is what it is and that there's got to be a way through it.

MICHAEL J. FOX

MANLY DISTRACTION

A lot of men are particularly good at ignoring their emotions, and I've often been guilty of trying to distract myself from mine. Whether it's alcohol, food, work, sex or even exercise, we all find things to help us cope with uncomfortable feelings. If I'm not busy doing something, I have to face myself, and I don't always like what I see. The issue is that most of these distractions are socially acceptable, so other men and women aren't concerned when they see a guy drinking regularly or eating too much, or working long hours. We need to become more aware of how we use these everyday activities as distractions from what's really going on inside.

MENTAL HEALTH AS A CONTINUUM

If we imagine mental health as a continuum, with feeling absolutely terrible at one end and feeling on top of the world at the other, most people will sit somewhere in the middle of the line, and they will likely move around. It's not the case that you're either depressed or not depressed. It's much more complex and less black and white than that.

Your emotional state can change from one moment to the next, and you can feel great in one area of your life and terrible in another. There are no rules! When I realized that my issues were not all-encompassing and made up of only one factor, it was a great relief to me, as I could compartmentalize the areas that I was struggling with, which then made tackling them more viable. It helped me to move on from being labelled as "depressed" or "anxious" by doctors based on a rudimentary questionnaire.

Remember that your personal situation is more complex and unique than the label it might be given, so your solution will also likely be unique.

MOOD

MENTALLY ILL	LANGUISHING	MENTALLY HEALTHY	FLOURISHING
• Depressed mood • Socially withdrawn • Poor sleep	• Stuck • Feeling empty • Low vitality	• Satisfied • Feel valued • Generally positive	• Thriving • Self-accepting • Meaning in life

TURN YOUR FACE TO THE SUN

AND THE SHADOWS FALL BEHIND YOU.

MAORI PROVERB

SUICIDAL THOUGHTS

According to WHO, a person dies every 40 seconds from suicide. Suicide is the biggest killer of men under 45 in the UK, and men are three times more likely to die from suicide than women, according to current statistics from Samaritans (part of the international charity network Befrienders Worldwide).

In many parts of the world suicide rates are worsening – in the US the rate increased by 25 per cent between 1999 and 2016 according to the Centers for Disease Control and Prevention. There are so many things to fear in this world that can kill us, and yet statistically, in the younger part of our lives, the thing we should most be afraid of is ourselves.

I've had suicidal thoughts, but actually going through with it – that's quite another thing. The potential impact on friends and family has always stopped me from having more than just thoughts. But it's amazing how many others will admit to having had similar thoughts and feelings.

An audit from CALM (Campaign Against Living Miserably) in 2015 suggested that more than four in ten men under the age of 45 in the UK have contemplated taking their own lives. Life can have huge ups and downs, so it's understandable, at some point, to feel like you can't go on. Suicide is currently something of a taboo subject, but one that we – especially men – must begin to speak about more openly if we are to tackle the problem. See chapter 5 if you are feeling suicidal and need help urgently.

THE DANGER
OF ISOLATION

Research shows that social isolation is a major contributor to depression. In my experience, when I feel down I withdraw socially which, ironically, makes me feel worse. This can become a vicious cycle of depression and isolation. I feel that I should be able to deal with my problems alone and will only re-emerge once I feel better about myself inside. But there is real danger in loneliness – as humans we need emotional sustenance from interactions with other people.

A survey commissioned by the Mental Health Foundation found that women are far more likely to reach out to friends or family when suffering from a mental health issue. Isolation when struggling will only make the situation worse. We need to learn from the strong individuals in our societies who are open with their emotions and cope with life's challenges by connecting with others, not by shutting themselves off from the world.

"Two out of five men do not seek support when they need to because they prefer to solve their own problems."

Samaritans, 2019

THE HEALTH RISK OF SUPPRESSING EMOTIONS

It has been proven that bottling up your emotions may have negative impacts on both your mental and physical health, and consequently could affect every area of your life. If you don't deal with the emotions that you're feeling, your mind and body may not be able to take the impact of the stress. It might be possible to end up with mental health issues such as anxiety or depression, and physical health issues such as diabetes, heart disease or cancer according to research published in the US Journal of Psychosomatic Research. Stress causes inflammation in the body and inflammation can lead to illness. Surely that's reason enough to open up. As worrying as these research findings are, they inspire me to have vulnerable conversations about how I'm feeling. Hopefully they will inspire you, too.

"Forty-four per cent of men say they suppress their emotions often or at least once a day."

YouGov, 2017

I HAVE LEARNED NOW THAT WHILE THOSE WHO SPEAK ABOUT ONE'S MISERIES USUALLY HURT,

THOSE WHO KEEP SILENCE HURT MORE.

C. S. LEWIS

FINDING THE RIGHT KIND OF HELP

Realizing you need some help with your mental health is the biggest step to feeling better. Admitting to myself, and those around me, that I needed some help enabled me to start the journey of learning how to manage my emotions. Don't be discouraged or disheartened if you don't find the right professional help straight away. The lists for public mental health services can be long.

Currently, in the UK National Health Service, there is a maximum 18-week waiting time – that is an extremely long time if you're in a dark place. Private healthcare can get you seen more quickly but, as with the US private healthcare system, of course there are cost implications. I was given a three- to four-month expected waiting time to see a public specialist in the UK, so I decided to pay for private care. However, there are free services out there where you can get immediate help, which are detailed in chapter 5. The key is to persevere with your efforts and stay focused on getting the help you need.

Twenty-five times more is spent on research into cancer than mental health per person affected.

MQ UK MENTAL HEALTH RESEARCH FUNDING REPORT 2014–2017

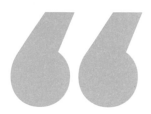

Don't be afraid to ask for help when you need it... Asking for help isn't a sign of weakness, it's a sign of strength.

CHAPTER 2

WHAT IS MENTAL HEALTH?

We all have mental health, just as we all have physical health. Sometimes our bodies are in good shape and sometimes they're not – the same can apply to our minds. It's important to understand the common causes of mental health issues, as well as the different types of mental health issues, so that we can treat ourselves in the right way to feel better. Self-care treatment methods are explored in chapter 4, but it's important to seek professional advice if you are struggling for more than a couple of weeks without any signs of improvement.

WHAT MENTAL HEALTH NEEDS IS MORE SUNLIGHT,

MORE CANDOUR, MORE UNASHAMED CONVERSATION.

FACTORS THAT CONTRIBUTE TO MENTAL HEALTH ISSUES

So what are the kinds of things in life that cause us to have mental health difficulties? Nature and nurture both play a part. Here are some of the main causes:

> **Major stressful life situations, such as financial troubles, death of a loved one or relationship break-ups**

> **Having a blood relative with a mental illness**

> **Having few close friends or healthy relationships**

> **Traumatic experiences, such as being abused, assaulted or bullied**

> **Having a chronic medical condition**

UNDERSTANDING PAST TRAUMAS

For me, a major trauma that I went through was being bullied at school. Being bullied in my teenage years gave me a massive rejection complex. As humans, we all want acceptance and love, but this was the opposite of what I received at school for those two formative years.

We all go through difficulties in our lives; simply identifying those difficulties and taking a step back from them is the first action on the road to managing their impact. Understanding that there was a cause for the way I felt was a huge relief, as it helped me to speak with others about it and realize that it wasn't my fault.

So, it can be helpful to dig into your earlier life experiences with a view to comprehending how they may have shaped the way that you see the world now. Friends and family members can be useful sounding boards for these investigations, but a trained mental health professional will likely be able to help you find answers more effectively. It's important to recognize that everyone experiences some level of trauma in their lives, so don't dwell on your past trauma; rather, use the awareness to improve your present and future.

STRESS, ANXIETY AND DEPRESSION ARE CAUSED WHEN WE ARE LIVING TO PLEASE OTHERS.

PAULO COELHO

FEELING LOW

It's important to note that you don't have to be diagnosed with a mental health disorder to justify how you feel. Perhaps you generally feel down, helpless, different or a bit worthless. This is all totally OK. I believe that mental health disorders are not an exact science – as previously mentioned, each of them is on a continuum from mild to severe and it's totally possible to be suffering with elements of a few disorders without being diagnosed as being so. Your experience is simply that: it's yours. The key thing is to identify how you feel and then figure out the best way to reach out for the help you need – that might be through talking to a friend, self-care (see Chapter 4) or speaking to a therapist.

THE MAIN MENTAL HEALTH CONDITIONS

ANXIETY

Anxiety is a state of excessive worry and is normally focused on potential (negative) future outcomes. Of course, worry is a totally normal emotion that all of us will experience throughout our lives, but it becomes a problem when the worry lasts for a long time and our fears are not relative to the size of the problems we face. This can prevent you from living a normal life, making you avoid certain situations where your worries might become distressing and hard to control. Anxiety can result in a panic attack – heart pounding, struggling to breathe, legs shaking, hot and cold sweats or feeling light-headed. In a moment like this, it's important to let others know that you are feeling anxious and explain your symptoms, so that they can support you.

An example of anxiety

Although I had experienced anxiety since my teenage years, the first time I recognized it as anxiety was during my last year of university. I was constantly worrying about my next steps – getting a job and starting my career. I remember buying a book called *How to Stop Worrying and Start Living*, as the title resonated strongly with how I was feeling. I couldn't stop my brain from overthinking and catastrophizing my life. This affected my sleep, self-esteem, motivation and desire to socialize.

Since then, the anxiety has shown up throughout my life, mainly around work, friends and relationships. Learning how to manage my anxious thoughts has been a challenging journey and perhaps one I will always be on, but it is absolutely possible to do so with the right support and self-care.

That the birds of worry and care fly over your head, this you cannot change, but that they build nests in your hair, this you can prevent.

CHINESE PROVERB

PHOBIAS

Phobias are the most common anxiety disorder. They are triggered by a specific situation or object, despite there being no actual danger. Common phobias are of spiders, heights or flying, but you could have an irrational fear of literally anything. A more modern phobia is being without, or not being able to use, your mobile phone – nomophobia. It's totally normal to have fears about particular objects or situations. However, according to the Diagnostic and Statistical Manual of Mental Disorders, a fear becomes a phobia when your feelings aren't relative to the danger you're in and these feelings last for more than six months. When phobias are severe they can become debilitating, but the good news is that almost all phobias can be treated and managed. If you find that yours is having an impact on the way you live your life, consider speaking to your GP.

DEPRESSION

Depression is a low mood that lasts for at least a couple of weeks or reoccurs for a few days at a time and affects your everyday life. It can range from mild depression, where you're consistently in low spirits, to severe, where you're suicidal. From my personal experience, I'd say it feels like everything in normal life is difficult and not worthwhile, and it feels impossible to enjoy the things that you normally would take pleasure in.

You might feel like isolating yourself from other people, not bothering with the activities you'd usually take part in and find yourself questioning whether life is worth living. It's critical at those times to remind yourself that you may be suffering from an illness, a mental disease; and as with most physical diseases, you can manage it and recover.

I found that with depression, one of the most important things you could realize is that you're not alone.

DWAYNE JOHNSON AKA "THE ROCK"

EATING DISORDERS

Food is a surprisingly common thing to use to express our feelings. For example, we might over-eat or under-eat when we're having difficulty with our mental health. Diagnosing this use of food to handle emotions as an eating disorder requires analysis of your eating patterns as well as medical tests of your weight, blood and body mass index (BMI). The main eating disorders are anorexia, bulimia and binge eating, but the way your relationship with food impacts on your mental health might not necessarily fit into any one category. According to the National Centre for Eating Disorders, men only account for approximately five to ten per cent of eating disorder sufferers, but this can be as high as fifty per cent in younger sufferers. Most go undiagnosed due to a reluctance to seek treatment.

POST-TRAUMATIC STRESS DISORDER (PTSD)

PTSD is a type of anxiety disorder which can develop anytime from immediately to years after experiencing a traumatic event. It has mainly been used to describe the symptoms of anxiety that war veterans exhibit, but it's now recognized that a wide range of traumatic experiences can result in PTSD. There are a variety of symptoms, from hypervigilance to a patchy memory of the event and generally feeling unsafe with no reason to be so.

The trauma of being bullied may have given me symptoms of PTSD. I have struggled to trust people and allow them to get close to me, always keeping people at arm's length and struggling to express affection. I have always had to keep busy, constantly distracting myself with the next thing, and the next thing... Seeking help has enabled me to understand the trauma better and accept that it's not my fault; rather, it is a consequence of something that was out of my control. We all go through some degree of trauma in our lives, which won't necessarily lead to PTSD, but it's worth having an understanding of the disorder, should you recognize symptoms in yourself or others.

PSYCHOSIS

Psychosis can be a symptom of many mental disorders such as schizophrenia, bipolar disorder or severe depression. It is when you perceive reality in a very different way to those around you. This might be hearing voices, seeing things that other people don't hear or see, or having false beliefs that no one else shares, such as thinking that you can control the weather. These experiences can be extremely frightening and of course you should ask for immediate support from those around you and seek professional medical help.

OBSESSIVE-COMPULSIVE DISORDER (OCD)

In OCD, the "obsessive" refers to undesirable thoughts, worries and doubts that come into your mind and make you feel mentally uncomfortable or anxious. The "compulsive" refers to the fact that you feel compelled to do certain things to reduce this mental discomfort, such as repeatedly checking that a door is locked or that you turned the gas cooker off. People with OCD recognize that this behaviour is irrational, but they can't stop themselves from acting on their compulsions.

When I was at school, I remember having to touch objects such as a chair or wall within a certain timeframe, for fear that something bad would happen to my family if I didn't. These days, I have a much more common OCD around double- or triple-checking that doors and windows are locked, despite having locked the door myself only moments before. This is a surprisingly common disorder, but usually manageable with the right help. It's important to recognize it for what it is and seek help if it starts to disrupt your day-to-day life.

If there are three cans in the fridge, he'll throw one away because it has to be an even number.

VICTORIA BECKHAM ON DAVID'S OCD

FIGHT OR FLIGHT

Many mental health disorders can leave us feeling like we are in danger, and our bodies react to this perceived danger just as they did hundreds of years ago when we had more physical threats to deal with – by triggering the urge either to run away or to fight. When you perceive that you are under threat, your body releases hormones like adrenaline and cortisol, which speed up your heart rate and make you more alert. This is great if you've just spotted a lion on the horizon, but not so good if you've just remembered something negative that someone said to you as a child or an email has just arrived from your boss. You can end up in a constant state of alertness, which takes its toll on your mind and body, so you need to learn how to manage this stress response by adopting self-care practices that work for you.

IT'S NOT STRESS THAT KILLS US,

IT IS OUR REACTION TO IT.

HANS SELYE

NEGATIVE COPING MECHANISMS

There are many ways that people cope and get on with life while suffering from mental health issues. The problem is that the easiest coping mechanisms are often short-term solutions and detrimental to mental health. What is more, these coping strategies are usually socially acceptable and some are even celebrated. Below are some of the most common; you may well find that you can identify with at least one of them. Consider how you might be using these to avoid facing your feelings.

> Alcohol

> Overeating or undereating

> Smoking

> "Retail therapy"

> Caffeine

> Work

> Sex

> Busyness

> Isolation

> Gambling

YOUR MENTAL HEALTH IS UNIQUE

There are other types of mental health conditions, as well as the most common ones described in this chapter, so, if you think your problem is at the more serious end of the spectrum, it's worth seeking professional support to get a proper diagnosis.

Having said that, it's really important to recognize that your mental health is unique – you may be experiencing elements of different conditions at the same time. As humans we like to put things and people into "boxes", so that they are easier to understand and deal with, but there is no one on this planet who has the exact same nature (and nurture) as you. So use the support of professionals who understand these conditions, but recognize that your situation cannot be compared to that of anyone else.

CHAPTER 3

NORMALIZING MENTAL HEALTH

To get men talking about mental health we need to break down the stigmas associated with it. We need to try to accept how we feel, open up about our emotions and encourage our friends to do the same. There is huge power in vulnerability and that power is in your hands, should you choose to use it.

Everything can be taken from a man but one thing: the last of the human freedoms – to choose one's attitude in any given set of circumstances, to choose one's own way.

VIKTOR E. FRANKL

ACCEPTANCE

It's vital to accept how you feel in order to make progress with your problem. If you feel low, recognize that and accept it in the present moment. Maybe you don't want to feel the way you do, but resisting how you feel will only make it worse, as you will be suppressing a totally normal human emotion.

Things go wrong in everyone's life, and at times everyone feels bad. If you can accept how you feel right now, without resistance, you stand a much greater chance of feeling better sooner. This is easier said than done, but it's worth really trying to feel your emotion. I find that simply sitting still and turning my attention toward my body helps me to get in touch with how I feel. Perhaps meditation will work for you, or journalling, or telling a friend. Feel it and accept it.

"Happiness cannot forever be sustained... It's a transitory thing."

Russell Brand

NO QUICK FIX, BUT YOU CAN MANAGE

I've tried an enormous number of therapies and techniques – everything from cognitive behavioural therapy to cold-water swimming – but I've found nothing has been a quick fix for my mental health struggles. They are part of who I am. However, there are many techniques and people that you can turn to, and from them you can devise your own toolkit to help you tackle issues as they arrive. I've accepted that my anxiety might not go away; that, for now, it is a part of my life, as it is for many other men. The focus needs to be on how best to manage it, on a daily, hourly and moment-by-moment basis.

REALIZE
DEEPLY THAT
THE PRESENT
MOMENT
IS ALL YOU
EVER HAVE.

ECKHART TOLLE

A deeply personal experience

No other person can fully understand what you are going through – not your partner, your best friend or your family. If you do try to explain it to them (which I'd highly recommend), they will have their own perception of what you tell them. Your experience of your mental health is simply that: it's yours. It's 100 per cent subjective. So there's no point comparing your situation to that of others, or expecting others to understand completely what you're going through. The best that they can do is to support you.

THE WORLD ULTIMATELY IS

WHAT WE SAY IT IS.

DAVID FRIEDRICH STRAUSS

For me the most important aspect to keeping your mental health in check is to be open and honest about how you feel with the people around you.

DR ALEX GEORGE

BE THE ROLE MODEL

The men who are most revered in society, whether powerful, successful, wealthy or famous, are, for the most part, not likely to admit their mental health struggles in public, which leaves us regular guys feeling uncertain about opening up and speaking out.

However, thankfully, this seems to be changing. With the likes of Thierry Henry, Tyson Fury and Princes Harry and William getting involved in the debate, the tide is turning. But we don't have to wait for others to open up before we do so ourselves. I still struggle to open up, but every time I do my relationships deepen and the burden of my anxiety eases. What's more, I relieve the burden of someone else – we're all carrying it to some degree.

If we could change ourselves, the tendencies in the world would also change. As a man changes his own nature, so does the attitude of the world change towards him.

GANDHI

Walk and talk

Hopefully you can understand the benefits of opening up about your feelings to those around you, but in practice it can seem quite daunting to do it. Perhaps start by opening up to one person – someone close to you whom you can spend some time with alone. You may find, as I do, that sitting opposite someone (even if you know them well) can feel quite intense and not conducive to discussing feelings. If so, you might find it much easier to talk about how you're feeling while going for a walk. It's less scary to tell someone you're struggling when they're not staring you in the eyes! Obviously phone calls or messages can also be great ways of sharing your thoughts, but it's much easier to connect with someone when you're physically with them.

NO MAN IS AN ISLAND, ENTIRE OF ITSELF;

EVERY MAN IS A PIECE OF THE CONTINENT, A PART OF THE MAIN.

JOHN DONNE

CONNECT AND COMMUNICATE

Humans are hyper-social animals. Everything we think, feel and do is influenced by our social experiences, so it's critical that we connect with other people. I often completely withdraw and disconnect from other people when I feel low. My family can easily tell when I'm down, as I simply don't contact them; or if I do, I do it in the briefest way possible.

Men in particular can struggle with social connection in times of difficulty, perhaps because of the social stereotyping about how men should behave. So don't disconnect, but recognize your tendency to not want to express yourself when you're feeling low. Figure out how you best connect and with whom.

On the occasions that I do share how I'm feeling, the response is always supportive, without exception. The more I share, the easier it becomes and the more normal I feel because so many others have similar struggles. With a more open dialogue around mental health we can together make discussing your emotions as easy as talking about the weather.

There will be good people around you, good souls wanting to help. Even when it seems impossible to open our mouths... we must.

FEARNE COTTON

Keep an eye on your friends

We all know it's good to look out for your friends, but more than buying your buddy a drink, it's really important to learn how to spot the signs of mental health difficulties. Perhaps a friend of yours has been drinking a lot more than normal recently, isolating himself from your friendship group or acting out of character. Ask how he is and don't accept "I'm fine" as a response. Ask twice if you sense that he might not be and check how he's really doing. If he says he's struggling, don't be afraid to ask how low he feels.

If you think that someone is suffering to the extent of being a suicide risk, the UK mental health charity Mind advocates asking direct questions such as "Are you having suicidal thoughts?" and, if so, "Have you made any plans?". Research in the United States has found that asking people who are suicidal about their thoughts doesn't make them any more likely to act on them. It's much better that you know and can support them than that they suffer in silence.

A REAL FRIEND IS ONE WHO WALKS IN WHEN THE REST OF THE WORLD WALKS OUT.

WALTER WINCHELL

THINGS TO SAY TO A FRIEND WHO'S STRUGGLING

When a friend opens up to you about struggling with his mental health, It's important to support him rather than try to resolve his issues. Men can be particularly direct in dealing with everyday problems, rushing to offer a practical solution, but mental health is such a personal experience that it's impossible to understand truly what someone is going through, and therefore extremely difficult to resolve.

Don't tell him to "toughen up" or "man up", or say it'll be alright or that you know how he feels. The most helpful way you can contribute is to listen and ask if there is anything you can do. Let him know that you care and want him to feel better. Suggest sources of support such as other friends, family or mental health services and offer your time to participate in his life. Maybe suggest doing something together that you know he enjoys.

CALM's Five Steps to Help a Friend:

1. Ask – encourage him to open up. Don't be afraid to use the word suicide.

2. Listen – listen without judgement.

3. Make a plan – create structure, set simple goals. If he is suicidal, stay with him and call emergency services.

4. Build a support squad – call in family and friends. Share details of helplines such as CALM and Samaritans.

5. Keep checking in – don't stop because you think he's better.

USE APPROPRIATE LANGUAGE

When asking a friend about mental health, it's helpful to tailor your questions to him, particularly if he hasn't discussed this kind of emotional stuff before. Perhaps rather than "How are you feeling?" you could ask "I've noticed that you're drinking more than normal; is everything OK?". Or instead of "Why are you isolating yourself?" you could ask "You haven't been hanging out with us recently – what's up?". We need to create new norms in language, where it's just as OK to talk about how we're feeling as it is to talk about sports.

OPENING UP AT WORK

As we spend approximately a third of our lives at work, the workplace environment plays an extremely important part in tackling the stigmas around mental health. A toxic environment can be corrosive to our mental health and a positive environment can give it a boost (as well as make us more productive workers).

Both employers and employees have a role to play in creating a work environment and culture that is conducive to constructive conversations about the mental health of all staff members. So whether you are at the top or bottom of your organization, you can take actions to enable others to open up; the easiest way to do this is to open up yourself, perhaps by having an honest conversation with someone in your team, whether more senior or junior than you. I have built really meaningful relationships with work colleagues through these kinds of chats, which have created a happier and more productive working environment.

"Only 13 per cent of people feel able to disclose a mental health issue to their line manager."

Mental Health at Work Report 2017

WHAT HAPPENS WHEN PEOPLE OPEN THEIR HEARTS?

THEY GET BETTER.

HARUKI MURAKAMI

THE POWER OF VULNERABILITY

Wanting or needing help is nothing to be ashamed of. Showing your true self with all of its imperfections is the simplest and most powerful way to drive the conversation about male mental health forward. As humans, we are made to connect with others; this is what gives our lives purpose and meaning. Contrary to our prevailing male culture, I have learned that sharing my perceived weaknesses draws people toward me, not away from me. The best friendships I have are those in which I have shared my whole self, not the self that I think others want to see. By being truly vulnerable with others we build trust and that is the foundation of connection, which we all need to have good mental health.

IMPERFECTIONS ARE NOT INADEQUACIES; THEY ARE REMINDERS THAT WE'RE ALL IN THIS TOGETHER.

BRENÉ BROWN

CHAPTER 4

SELF-CARE

Self-care means, quite literally, taking care of yourself, and it is important for everyone to do, regardless of their gender. There are things that we can all do to maintain and improve our mental health or fitness. But what's right for you will likely be different to what is right for others. Our experience of life is unique and so are the ways in which we deal with life's ups and downs. It's worth trying lots of different self-care methods to see what helps to boost your mood; then you will have a toolkit of things that you can integrate into your life as and when you need them.

Healthy body, healthy mind?

I spent the first 30 years of my life living by the "healthy body, healthy mind" philosophy. I assumed that if I ate the right food and exercised, I'd not only have good physical health, but I'd have good mental health, too. This didn't work on its own. Having a healthy body certainly helps to create the right conditions, but there is a lot more to mental well-being. The brain could be considered a muscle that you must keep well nourished and exercised in order for it to be healthy. Self-care could be considered the exercise for your mind.

AN EMPTY LANTERN PROVIDES NO LIGHT.

SELF-CARE IS THE FUEL THAT ALLOWS YOUR LIGHT TO SHINE BRIGHTLY.

ANONYMOUS

FIVE-A-DAY
FOR YOUR BRAIN

WHO tells us to eat at least five portions of fruit and vegetables per day and exercise for at least 150 minutes per week to keep our bodies physically healthy and prevent disease. Why don't we do the same for our minds? Simple day-to-day behaviours such as walking in nature, acts of gratitude or journalling your thoughts can have a profound impact on how you feel.

For the first of my mental five-a-day, I try to get outdoors early in the morning. It really makes me feel better, probably because fresh air lowers levels of cortisol (the stress hormone) in the body. Every day is different, but I might also meditate, connect with a friend, play a game of squash, do ten minutes of yoga or practise a moment of mindfulness while doing a routine task such as hanging up the washing. Simple habits are the key to good health, both physically and mentally.

Get into nature

The times I spent messing around in the woods near the house where I grew up are some of my fondest memories – I'm always drawn to nature, particularly when I feel anxious or depressed. This could be explained by "biophilia" – which is a hypothesis that humans possess an innate attraction to nature, resulting from our biological connection with it.

Nature is non-judgemental, present and simply healing. Scientifically speaking, being surrounded by the natural environment has the power to decrease activity in the prefrontal cortex, which is the brain region where rumination takes place.

"I need nature. It makes me realize that all of this was here millions of years before me, and it'll be here millions of years after I'm gone. Something about that really helps put my problems into perspective."

Jake Tyler, mental health advocate

LOOK DEEP INTO NATURE AND THEN YOU WILL UNDERSTAND EVERYTHING BETTER.

ALBERT EINSTEIN

DARK THOUGHTS

We all have difficult, dark thoughts crossing our minds at some point – some will have these on a more recurring basis than others. This is totally OK – dark thoughts are like great thoughts, in the sense that they are only thoughts. They are not real; they are not you. They do not represent who you are or what you want.

We are predisposed to overthinking as a result of our prefrontal cortex, which is larger and more developed in humans than in any other organism; this is the part of the brain responsible for remembering, planning, decision-making and problem-solving. So recognize that your brain is a wonderfully powerful thing that sometimes gets a bit carried away.

NOTHING CAN HARM YOU AS MUCH AS

YOUR OWN THOUGHTS UNGUARDED.

BUDDHA

PHYSICAL ACTIVITY

Physical activity has a direct impact on your mental well-being. One of the easiest ways to boost your mood is to do some exercise. Research shows that feel-good chemicals called endorphins are released in the brain when you're active. But this doesn't have to mean running like you're training for a marathon – any kind of movement of your body that uses your muscles and expends energy can do the trick. I even find that simple stretching when I get out of bed in the morning can help me to reduce my levels of anxiety and make facing the day more achievable.

GENTLE EXERCISE

Depression is linked to the sedentary lifestyles that people are increasingly living in the modern world, where technology removes so much of our day-to-day labour. Exercise in the contemporary sense wasn't necessary when you had to grow your own food or walk everywhere. But exercise is simply moving your body to sustain or improve your health and fitness and we can take lessons from the forms of exercise that our ancestors did without labelling it as exercise. It doesn't have to be intense to reap the benefits. Any kind of exercise is useful, as long as it suits you and you do enough of it. Ideally, it's something that you enjoy and fits into your daily life, so that you can do it regularly and with ease. This could be as simple as taking the stairs instead of the lift, walking or cycling to work, gardening or doing any kind of manual labour around the house.

INTENSE EXERCISE

If you feel up to it, high-intensity exercise can have significant benefits for your mental health in a very short period of time. Whether it's sprinting for a short distance, doing as many push-ups as you can in one minute or following a 20-minute high-intensity interval training (HIIT) workout video, it's possible to boost your mental well-being in a brief spell of concerted effort.

If you're time-poor, integrating a HIIT workout into your day is a great option to lift your spirits. I have found that simply doing ten quick press-ups every day gives me a bit of this mood lift. It's really fast and can be done anywhere, so there's no reason not to do it. Why not put down this book and try something right now to see if it works for you?

Do "pointless" things

In our competitive, global world where technology constantly updates us on the lives of others, we can feel that everything we do must have a reason to it. Perhaps we must learn something, achieve something or impress others with our actions. There is almost always a goal in mind. But there is great value for our mental health in doing so-called "pointless" things – that is, things that have no desired outcome other than the moment-by-moment enjoyment of doing them. How could you reclaim your childlike playfulness and ability to do something solely for the sake of doing it? It could be lying on your back spotting cloud shapes or doodling on a piece of paper destined for the trash. Be there in that moment and don't try to achieve anything from what you're doing.

COMMUNITY

A sense of community can really help to ward off poor mental health and drive positive well-being. Feeling part of something bigger than ourselves makes us think more about others, and it takes us out of our own heads. We are social animals and need connection with other human beings to survive. Community can be found through family, friends, neighbours, hobbies, sports or literally anything that gets people together.

If I'm feeling low, I find it's easier to be part of communities where I can spend time with other people but not have to talk too much, such as sports clubs. If you're not feeling well, going out for a meal with friends or to a party with lots of people can feel overwhelming. If you're really struggling to connect with people in person, keeping in touch through social media, messaging or email can also help to give you a sense of community in the short term.

However, it's important to remember that real-world connections are far more beneficial for our mental health than virtual connections; studies show that too much time spent online can actually increase mental health disorders, such as anxiety and depression, so make sure you get balance.

WE CANNOT LIVE ONLY FOR OURSELVES.

A THOUSAND FIBRES CONNECT US WITH OUR FELLOW MEN.

HENRY MELVILL

SLEEP

Sleep is just as important as what we eat and drink. It restores and repairs the body, and allows the brain to consolidate memories and process information, which enables us to function effectively during the daytime. Sleep and mental health are inextricably linked, and research shows that a lack of sufficient sleep is linked to psychological distress. So a healthy sleep routine is key – have a regular bedtime and wake-up time, remove digital devices from the bedroom, get some exercise during the day and avoid stimulants close to bedtime. Bed should be for sleep and sex only – if you are awake for more than 20 minutes, get up until you feel sleepy again.

Insomnia is something that I really struggle with – anxiety loves to rear its ugly head in the early hours – but I find that getting up and getting on with the day is the best way to deal with it. Figure out what kind of sleep schedule works for you. It doesn't have to be eight hours, in one go, between 11 p.m. and 7 a.m. According to Harvard Medical School, there can be some substantial differences among individuals' sleep requirements, with varying circadian rhythms and genetic predispositions. We're all unique and our specific rest requirements are also unique; so don't beat yourself up if your sleep pattern doesn't fit with some societal convention.

MASSAGE

A great way to boost your mood could be to have a massage; whether it's from a proper massage therapist or your partner/friend. Studies show that massage greatly reduces mental illness symptoms by increasing blood circulation. This enables an increase in dopamine, which is the hormone associated with feeling happy. From the human touch there can also be a release of oxytocin, which is regarded as the love hormone as it gives a sense of belonging and trust. For me, massages are a very lazy way to help me relax; I find that after a really firm massage I can feel like I've done some exercise without even moving!

DECREASE STIMULANTS

It's likely no surprise that alcohol, caffeine and sugar aren't good for your mental health. These are all stimulants that affect the central nervous system and cause inflammation in the body. They may make us feel more alert or more relaxed in the short term but will always have negative effects on mood in the long term. Alcohol can be a particularly tough one to reduce. It's hard to be the guy who orders a soft drink when all your friends are buying rounds of beer. But your brain will thank you for it if you can stay strong and drink less. Life is too short to follow the crowd when you know it's going to make you feel bad.

MEDITATION AND MINDFULNESS

I find it's really hard to relax when I'm feeling low. You don't feel motivated to do anything, yet you can't relax while doing nothing. It's a horrible feeling, but it's one that you can only get yourself out of by doing something. If you don't feel like moving, that something could be meditation, which is scientifically proven to reduce symptoms of depression and anxiety. Meditation doesn't mean you have to sit still with your legs crossed for hours; simply get into a comfortable position, close your eyes and focus on your breath as it enters and leaves your nose. Even doing so for two minutes is long enough to feel the benefits.

Personally, I prefer mindfulness meditation, which is paying attention to the present moment with non-judgement. You could do this while walking to the shops or eating your lunch. Each time you notice that your mind has wandered to a thought, gently bring it back to what you're doing. This should help to stop the ruminations that keep you feeling down. But remember that meditation can come in many forms – sport works particularly well for me, as it focuses my mind on the present moment and doesn't allow me to think about anything else. Figure out what your version of meditation is.

"Understanding that the brain is a misunderstood tool and that we all come from a much deeper place has changed my whole perspective on life. Meditation gives me the space to detach from the volatile, autonomous mind and allow things to settle and just be as they are."

Ed Stafford, explorer and adventurer

MEDITATION IS NOT A WAY OF MAKING YOUR MIND QUIET.

IT'S A WAY OF ENTERING INTO THE QUIET THAT'S ALREADY THERE.

DEEPAK CHOPRA

THE POWER
OF THE BREATH

Breathing can be an extremely powerful tool to help us become calm and centred and as we spend our entire lives breathing, it's easy to assume that we know how to do it effectively. But often when we feel stress it becomes choppy, quick and shallow, and we end up in a cycle of stress causing shallow breathing and shallow breathing causing stress. This sets off the sympathetic nervous system, priming us for activity and response. If you can focus on your breath and slow it down, breathing fully and deeply, you can bring balance to your mind and body.

Breathing from your abdomen, with the belly expanding and the chest not rising, is called diaphragmatic breathing and is performed by all mammals when they are in a state of relaxation. If you watch a baby breathe, you'll see this in action. We can each create this state of relaxation by adopting this original breathing technique. Personally, I find that three really deep, slow breaths from the abdomen are enough to calm me down in a moment of panic.

GROUNDING

Research in the Journal of Environmental and Public Health suggests that putting the body in direct or uninterrupted contact with the earth can have a whole host of health benefits, one of which is reducing stress. Research is starting to show that modern humans' lack of contact with the earth is a contributing factor to many of the health problems we face today, and that grounding can have a positive effect on mood.

The theory is that you can "earth" your body in the same way as an electrical appliance, allowing excess positively charged particles to run off into the ground. If you've ever felt good walking barefoot on sand or grass, then this could well be a result of your positive charge being neutralized. So next time you're feeling overwhelmed with life, try kicking off your shoes and standing in direct contact with the earth and see if you can feel your body regaining balance. It might work for you, or it might not, but you won't know unless you try.

DO SOMETHING

It's totally normal to feel demotivated when you feel down, but when you procrastinate and put off making decisions it only makes you feel worse. So do something constructive – it doesn't matter what it is, but doing something is better than ruminating on how bad you feel. This isn't to say that you shouldn't accept how you feel, because that will help, but that you are more likely to feel better if you take action. This could be as simple as walking to the shops, talking to a neighbour, making some tea, putting the washing on or doing some work; anything to get you out of your head.

HABIT LINKS

When you find self-care activities that work for you, it's helpful to link those activities to existing habits in your normal day. This will greatly improve the likelihood of you regularly doing the things that make you feel better. For example, I have the habit of drinking tea every single day, and I find mindfulness a useful form of self-care. So, as I boil the kettle, I take a moment to practise some mindfulness, bringing my awareness to my surroundings – watching the steam come out of the kettle, noticing the tea slowly diffuse into the water and the smell rising up from the mug. It's imbedded into my routine, so most of the time I remember to do it, which easily creates the conditions for long-term improvement to my well-being.

DEPENDING ON WHAT THEY ARE, OUR HABITS WILL EITHER MAKE US OR BREAK US.

WE BECOME WHAT WE REPEATEDLY DO.

SEAN COVEY

DIET

It's now widely recognized that what we eat and drink can affect our mental state. Research is showing a two-way link between the nervous and gut systems, which perhaps should be no surprise if you've ever had an upset stomach when you're nervous about an exam or presentation. Eating a healthy diet will give your gut the nutrition it needs to keep both your body and mind in good shape.

This diet will be different for everyone, so when you're trying to eat more nutritious foods it's important to listen to your body's response to the fuel you're giving it. Check in and see how you feel during eating, straight after and hours later. We are all different so there is no one-size-fits-all diet. Work out what makes you feel best and try to make food choices on that basis. You won't be able to stick to it all the time, so don't beat yourself up for that. I work on an 80/20 rule; that is, if I can eat well for 80 per cent of the time, I'm giving myself a pretty good chance of feeling healthy, while not making my life a diet-controlled hell.

ONE CANNOT
THINK WELL,
LOVE WELL,
SLEEP WELL,
IF ONE HAS
NOT DINED
WELL.

VIRGINIA WOOLF

AFFIRMATIONS

Positive affirmations can encourage us to keep going when times are tough and we're struggling with our mental health. Simply having a positive sentence displayed above your desk, on your bathroom mirror or on your phone background can help you to calm down when you're feeling panicked or sad. Neuroscience research suggests that repeatedly using affirmations may have the power to rewrite the subconscious mind and enhance well-being.

By simply reading a few positive words and perhaps saying them out loud to yourself, you may be able to build resilience and overcome your negative thinking patterns. You need to find a sentence that resonates with you. I have "I am enough" above my desk to soothe me when I'm in a period of anxiety, perhaps thinking that I haven't been successful enough or worrying what people think of me.

Some more examples of positive affirmations are:

> My imperfections make me unique.

> I am worthy of love.

> I possess all the qualities I need to be successful.

> I choose to be happy.

> I am healthy and happy.

SO MANY OF OUR DREAMS AT FIRST SEEM IMPOSSIBLE, THEN THEY SEEM IMPROBABLE,

AND THEN, WHEN WE SUMMON THE WILL, THEY SOON BECOME INEVITABLE.

CHRISTOPHER REEVE

FIND YOUR QUIET SPACE

Taking time out in a quiet space in your home can be a powerful way to recharge. In today's frantic world, where we're rushing around and so often connected to other people, be that physically or technologically, it's difficult to disconnect for some downtime. Whether it's a garage or spare room or any space you can find to be alone, retreating when you feel a bit depleted can rejuvenate you so that when you re-emerge you're in a better headspace to handle the world again.

For me, as bizarre as it may sound, my quiet space is the toilet. It's a place I can lock the door literally and metaphorically on the outside world and take time to think. Could a designated quiet space be useful for you? Remember not to spend too much time in there if you're feeling low; it's helpful to have a bit of space, but it's not healthy to isolate yourself from other people for long periods of time, particularly when you're not feeling well.

LEARN FROM
THE LADIES

It may be that you need to challenge some of your preconceptions and stereotypical beliefs about what self-care looks like – perhaps by learning from the ladies in your life. Calming self-care activities like yoga or having a massage aren't defined by the gender you identify with. There is nothing "unmanly" about unwinding in a relaxing bubble bath at the end of a long day at work or practising daily meditation. I've recently joined a qigong group in which I'm the only man. Why not! What are the ladies in your life doing to look after themselves that you could learn from or join in with?

GET SOME PERSPECTIVE

When we feel down we tend to become very introspective, totally absorbed in our own problems, thoughts and situations. Getting yourself out of your own head can be a great way to alleviate a negative mood state, allowing you to focus on something bigger than yourself.

You could do this by asking how a friend or family member is feeling, taking an interest in the life of a vulnerable stranger or perhaps volunteering your time to help someone out. Getting some perspective on your own situation in the context of the society that you live in or the world that we share can be a powerful antidote in depressive times.

PERSPECTIVE IS EVERYTHING WHEN YOU ARE EXPERIENCING THE CHALLENGES OF LIFE.

JONI EARECKSON TADA

THE STRESS CONTAINER

Stress flows into our lives consistently and in many forms, whether it's work, family, money, and so on. This flow of stress fills up our internal "stress container", which can overflow if we don't find ways to release stress out of the bottom.

Self-care tools are ways to turn on the "tap" to let the stress out, and they need to be used consistently to ensure that the level in your stress container is kept manageable. Fill in the blanks for your own stressors and the self-care tools that could help you to ease them.

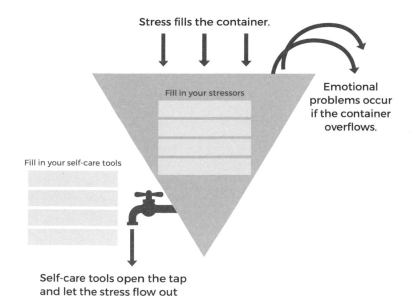

Stress fills the container.

Fill in your stressors

Emotional problems occur if the container overflows.

Fill in your self-care tools

Self-care tools open the tap and let the stress flow out

It's not the load that breaks you down; it's the way you carry it.

LOU HOLTZ

CHAPTER 5

GETTING PROFESSIONAL HELP

Sometimes you can manage your mental health yourself with self-care tools and the support of friends and family, but there could also be times when you need to get help from professionals who are trained to help people struggling. Recognizing that you need help is often the hardest step, but once you do it can feel like a huge weight off your shoulders. There is no shame in enlisting the support of someone who understands what you are going through.

PHYSICAL vs MENTAL

It's always helpful to think about your mental health in the same way as you do your physical health. If you had a common cold, you might give it a week or two for your body to get better and adjust your behaviour to help it do so, but if it didn't go away after a week or two you'd likely go to the doctor to get some professional advice.

Similarly, if you feel anxious for a couple of weeks, you might give yourself the time and self-care to improve, but if you don't improve you should seek support. Obviously, if physical or mental conditions are more severe, such as a broken leg or deep depression, you should seek out support urgently.

DO I NEED HELP?

It can be hard to know if and when you need professional help, particularly if you've never had any issues with your mental health before. Talking to a friend or family member about how you're feeling and asking their advice is a good place to start. If that feels too much, then simply writing down how you're feeling can help you to become a bit more aware of your emotional state.

So often we aren't in touch with what is going on inside of us, living in our heads and distracting ourselves with the outside world. I find journalling my thoughts really powerful – I forget grammar, punctuation and sentence structure and freely write down whatever is going on in my head. The process makes me more informed to change behaviours or seek help.

Free helplines

There are an ever-increasing number of free mental health services available to you, regardless of where you live in the world. Most countries have organizations that you can contact to get advice on how to get the help that you need. Searching on the Internet for support where you are will likely give you a range of options. For example, charities in the UK such as Mind and CALM and in the United States such as Mental Health America provide phone support, as well as online content to help you understand your situation better. There are even services that you can text for support such as Crisis Text Line in the United States and Shout in the UK.

SPEAK WITH YOUR DOCTOR

Your doctor's office is a great place to ask for help. It's confidential and doctors are trained to deal with your mental health as well as your physical health. You might be recommended to seek counselling or therapy, or perhaps to take some medication. As with any medical condition, it's important to take an active role in your treatment, questioning what you are advised in order to fully understand your treatment options. The treatment of mental health is much more complex, and arguably less comprehensively understood, than that of physical health. However, your doctor should certainly be made aware of your mental health, so have a chat and work out a strategy together.

Take your time healing, as long as you want. Nobody else knows what you've been through. How could they know how long it will take to heal you?

ANONYMOUS

WHAT TO DO
IN AN EMERGENCY

If you or someone you know is feeling suicidal, seek urgent support. You could go to the Emergency department of a hospital, call the Emergency Services or a crisis line number such as Samaritans (UK) on 116 123 and the National Suicide Prevention Lifeline (United States) on 1-800-273-8255, which are available 24 hours a day, 365 days a year.

CONCLUSION

We all have mental health and if, like me, you sometimes struggle with yours, remind yourself that it's totally normal. Life can be tough and your experience of it is totally unique, so the way that you will manage it will also be unique.

It's important to recognize that, as men, some of the ways that we have been traditionally socialized may not be conducive to good mental health. Not expressing ourselves and adopting unhealthy coping strategies to suppress how we really feel is not only damaging to ourselves but to society as a whole. We should consider adopting positive human traits rather than trying to adhere to traditional masculine or feminine stereotypes.

We all need to play our part in continuing to reduce the stigma around mental health, treating it just as seriously as physical health, increasing knowledge of the different types of disorders and being less black and white in our diagnoses of them. Opening up and showing vulnerability with your friends and family is the quickest and most effective way to improve your mental health and to show others that it's OK to do the same. Look out for your buddies. They, like me, might seem like they've got life all figured out while in reality on the inside they may be really struggling.

As much as the mental health issues I have dealt with, and continue to manage, have caused me great suffering, they have also taught me so many lessons. They have forced me to look inside myself for answers, rather than outside through external distractions, and continually to put the work into understanding who I really am. It's a journey, not a quick fix, and accepting where you are is the best place to start. Asking for professional help if you need it and building a self-care toolkit with healthy habits that you can build into your routine will set you up for a happier, healthier life.